FOOD 4 FAST FEET

by

Dr. Bala Naidoo

Cover design and graphics

by

John Mountain

TABLE OF CONTENTS

FOREWORD

Although I have been running for almost 40 years in Quebec and in British Columbia, I have to admit that I have not always paid enough attention to the nutritional aspects of running. This failure has a lot to do with the almost universal notion that when you are young, you think of yourself as being indestructible. However, as the years go by and you imperceptibly become an older runner, you begin to realize that the body does break down, especially if it is not well looked after.

Nutrition is one of the factors that play a vital role in helping to keep you running at your peak. What food to eat to keep your energy stores high and when to consume it to maximize that energy are important points to remember, whether you are an older or younger runner. So, if you want to keep running late into the sunset, you should pay attention to your nutrient and hydration needs at all times. This book attempts to show runners of all levels how to do it in simple language and without too much distraction from the underlying scientific rationale.

As you might imagine, this endeavour could be too onerous for one person to do all on his own. Fortunately, I had lots of help from many sources. I'll be remiss if I do not acknowledge the invaluable help and advice I received from my family and fellow runners. First, I have to thank my wife Pauline not only for ensuring that we eat sensibly but also that we stick to our regular training schedule. Our children Sarah, Robin, Loren and his wife Kara are all runners or exercise enthusiasts and we would like to think that our example had some bearing on their inclination for sports.

My wife and I could not have achieved our quite modest accomplishments in the running arena had it not been for the training, advice, encouragement and camaraderie of our running family from the Ladysmith Striders. I would particularly like to salute our Sunday runners Pauline Naidoo, Phil and Heather Howard, Chris Geens, Dolly Brown, John Mountain, Simon Timmer, Robin and David Billas, Bruce Youngren, David Van Horne, Gayla Hunter, Wade Richardson, Michelle Frazer, Terry

Morrow, Michael Rowell, Kim Judson, Harvey Khun Khun and Steve Sharp.

A special thank you to our good friend Dolly Brown for faithfully accompanying us on our long runs at our pace, even though she is a far more accomplished and speedier runner than we are. She also has the distinction of being a 105 lb pocket dynamo who averages a minimum of 80 km per week and is always ready to join anyone in a run, at any time of the day. Her glycogen stores seem to be always topped up but when does she find the time to eat?

We, on Vancouver Island, are lucky to have had incredible runners who blazed pathways on the running horizon for all of us and who now serve as beacons to our aspiring runners. I would include in this category some veteran runners like Maurice Tarrant and John Woodall of the Prairie Inn Harriers, Harry Thompson and Hazura Sangha of Ceevacs Running Club. Their exploits on the Vancouver Island Runners Association (VIRA) racing circuits and other venues are simply too numerous to mention. We who are runners owe them a tremendous debt of gratitude.

Dr Bala Naidoo
Ladysmith,
British Columbia

May 30, 2011

ACKNOWLEDGEMENTS

I would like to thank Kelly Schellenberg of Ceevacs Running Club for suggesting the name of this book, at a time when I was striving unsuccessfully for inspiration to come up with a catchy title.

Many thanks to Pauline Naidoo and John Mountain who kindly offered to proofread this book. Their criticisms and corrections are gratefully acknowledged. I take full responsibility for any remaining typos and other errors in the book.

A special thank-you to the talented John Mountain for using his artistry and technical wizardry to improve the appearance of this book beyond my wildest expectations.

FOOD **4** FAST FEET

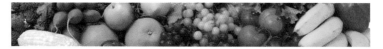

CHAPTER 1
GOOD NUTRITION IS CRITICAL
FOR GOOD PERFORMANCES

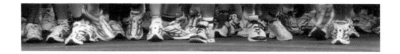

It is now recognized that nutrition is vitally important in determining running performance, delaying fatigue, speeding up the recovery process and even reducing running injuries. Unfortunately, many runners lack the necessary understanding of nutrition that would help them give their best. For example, eating too few calories will not give you enough energy to run at your peak but will instead make you feel tired as well as increasing the risk of injuries.

Although each one of us is different in terms of what foods we like to eat and what works best for us when we run, there are certain guidelines that can apply to all of us based on nutrition principles. For example, it is well known that fats are digested slowly by the body. So, if your breakfast is high in fat, it is likely to stay in your stomach for quite a while. If you run in the morning, having such a breakfast before a run is obviously not desirable.

A knowledge of nutrition is as important as knowing how to train for a particular race or event. After all, food is our fuel just as gasoline is that of cars. The more one runs, the more fuel the body requires. Any novice runner will quickly realize that in order to be able to run faster or longer, more and better types of food and fluids will be needed in addition to better training.

Eating the right food in the right amount and at the right time will not only help in providing you with the right amount of energy for your run but will also help repair damaged muscles in the recovery process after the run. Although your body will be using more carbohydrates, proteins and fats are also necessary. Many factors determine the relative amounts of these nutrients such as how fit you are, how long your run is and how fast you are running.

Once you get to know what you should be eating and drinking for optimum performance, you can then make the necessary changes in your diet that will help you, together with proper training, improve your running. In order to do that, a knowledge of the link between nutrition and energy production by the body is required.

First, the way you schedule your meals during the day may have to be modified. If you are like most of us, you probably work during the day, run after work and then come home for dinner. Your biggest meal is yet to come but you are banking on breakfast and lunch sustaining you during your run. However, unless you have had a high-energy snack before running, you'll probably find yourself running out of energy, especially if you're attempting a long run.

Does it make sense to have your big dinner after your run only to relax and then go to sleep?

It would be more sensible to have a big breakfast and lunch, together with snacks before your run, followed by a smaller dinner. In fact, by snacking often during the day, you'll maintain your blood sugar level and won't feel tired by the time you are ready to go for your run.

Remember to eat snacks that are low in fat and high in carbohydrate such as breakfast cereals, toast, energy bars, dried or fresh fruits. Your body will thus be adequately fuelled for your after-work run and a smaller dinner is enough to fuel your recovery.

As a rule we should be eating every 3 to 5 hours in order to keep our body fuelled up at all times and avoid big drops in blood sugar levels. This is why skipping meals is so bad for us. In fact, research has shown that instead of having three big meals in a day, it's better to split what you eat into four or five smaller meals.

No matter what changes you make, you should always start the day with a good breakfast loaded with carbohydrates to replenish your fuel level after sleeping.

Your main meals should also feature foods with lots of complex carbohydrates such as rice, pasta, potatoes, yams and beans. Complex carbohydrates release energy slowly and that's what you need on long runs.

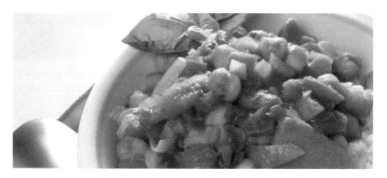

Runners in general need more food than sedentary people. For good nutrition, follow the Canada Food Guide in order to get the proper nutrients every day.

This means you should be consuming several servings of breads and grains followed by lots of vegetables and fruits, then some fish, meat, soy and dairy products with very little fat and sugar.

However, you should bear in mind that the Food Guide is designed for the average sedentary Canadian and the proportions given have to be tweaked in order to satisfy the requirements for runners.

For the average runner, running 1 km burns about 65 calories, so if you run 5 km a day, you'll need an extra 325 calories (5 x 65 calories) at least. Since regular running also increases your resting metabolism, you'll probably need around 400 extra calories per day.

If you do not increase the calories you eat by that amount, you'll lose weight and your running may suffer, unless you are overweight to start with. Eating a balanced diet with the right calorific intake and drinking adequate fluids are a must for runners.

As soon as you have finished running, you should start to refuel your body in order to restore the energy that you have spent, repair the minute muscle damages that have occurred and get you ready for your next run.

Fortunately, just after a run, the enzymes and hormones that have been used to ferry nutrients to your muscles during the run are most active. So, you should be eating plenty of carbohydrates and some protein as soon as possible, but at the most within the first hour after a run, to maximize absorption of these nutrients. This will not only help you to re-energize but will also help repair muscle damage that inevitably occurs when we run. This breaking and repairing action of muscles is what makes them eventually stronger.

We can break down our food into various components: carbohydrates, proteins, fats, vitamins, minerals, fibre, antioxidants and other phytonutrients. A healthy diet for the average runner should consist of about 60–65% carbohydrates, 20% protein and 20% fat. ♦

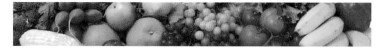

CHAPTER 2

CARBOHYDRATES

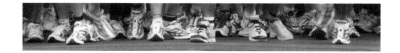

Carbohydrates are vital for runners as they are the primary fuel for all our muscular movements as well as being essential for our central nervous system and our brain.

All carbohydrates are broken down into glucose by the body. The body uses glucose for energy and any excess glucose is converted to glycogen, which is stored in the liver and muscles. When energy is needed by our muscles, glycogen can be converted back to glucose. About 5 grams of glucose, equivalent to 20 calories, stay in the bloodstream and is known as the blood sugar. Some of the glucose is also transported to the brain and other organs of the body.

Glucose in liver or muscles ⚙ glycogen (+ enzymes) ⚙ glucose

When we eat food several hours before a run, it will be digested and the carbohydrates converted to glucose and stored as glycogen. Right after eating, the blood glucose level rises. The hormone *insulin* is released from the pancreas to decrease the blood sugar. Insulin also carries glucose to muscles and speeds up the conversion of glucose to glycogen. Interestingly, it also stimulates muscle building and storage of body fat.

In reverse, another hormone, *glucagon*, is released when blood sugar is low and muscles are in need of energy. It spurs the liver to release glycogen which is converted to blood glucose.

How do we get the energy when we go for a run? At the start of a run, the muscles get their energy initially from their glycogen content. As we continue running, muscles absorb glucose, about 5 grams, present in the bloodstream. As running progresses, the blood glucose is used up and so more is released as glycogen from the liver. This ensures that the blood sugar does not fall too low.

An average male runner weighing about 68 kg(150 lb) and on a proper diet can store about 450 grams of muscle and liver glycogen. This will supply about 1800 calories or enough energy to run about 27 kilometres at a moderate pace. At this distance, he is likely to 'hit the wall' during a marathon (42.2 km), especially if he has not trained his body in using protein or fat as fuel. Extra energy in the form of a power drink or gel will also be needed in order to finish the marathon.

The body's ability to store glycogen is rather limited and it has to be refilled after vigorous exercise. Feeling tired and slowing down after a good start are signs that you are running low on glycogen. Rather than eating all your carbohydrate from a couple of big meals a day, divide it into several smaller portions and eat them every 3-5 hours to keep your energy high all day long.

It is interesting to note that although the body's glycogen storage is limited to about 1800 calories, the total body fat for an average 68 kg (150 lb) runner can potentially supply about 50 times more calories.

There are two kinds of carbohydrates: simple and complex ones. Both kinds yield glucose as their end product but they do so at different rates. Simple carbohydrates are found in refined sugars, jam, honey and other sweet foods and drinks made with sugar. These will be a quick source of glucose and should be consumed when you need energy quickly, that is just before a run, during a run and just after a run to fill up your depleted stores.

Most of your carbohydrate intake should, however, be focused on the nutrient-rich, complex ones which are found in high-fibre and unrefined foods such as fresh, starchy vegetables (carrots, peas, corn, potatoes, sweet potatoes) and fruits, whole grain cereals, porridge and multi-grained breads, brown rice and dried beans. Complex carbohydrates are digested more slowly than simple ones and provide energy over a longer period of time, a boon for distance runners.

CARBOHYDRATE REQUIREMENTS FOR RUNNING

The carbohydrate required to sustain lifestyle and running activities vary according to weight, distance and speed of the run. In general, a runner would need about 5 to 7 g per kilogram of body weight. The table below gives an approximate weight that has to be consumed per day.

CARBOHYDRATE REQUIRED PER Kg OF BODY WEIGHT					
Body weight in Kg or (lb)	Carbohydrate (g) per kg of body weight				
	4	5	6	7	8
50 (110)	200	250	300	350	400
59 (130)	236	295	354	413	472
68 (150)	272	340	408	476	544
77 (170)	308	385	462	535	616

Table 1

From Table 1, a 68 kg (150 lb) runner requiring 6g of carbohydrate per kilogram of body weight would need 408 g of carbohydrates per day.

CARBOHYDRATES BEFORE RUNNING

1. Eating a carbohydrate-loaded meal together with some protein and fat well before running (24 hours or longer) should result in the runner being well fuelled.

2. For a morning run, have a high carbohydrate breakfast 1-2 hours before. Include some protein but very little fat.

3. About 15 minutes before your run, you may want to ensure that your energy level is at a maximum by eating some simple carbohydrate such as a glucose candy.

CARBOHYDRATES WHILE RUNNING

1. Taking carbohydrate during a run will result in muscle glycogen not being depleted. The muscles thus get the required glucose from the bloodstream rather than from the stored energy. Running down glycogen stores in the muscles will cause muscle fatigue, thus slowing down the runner.

2. So, what kind of carbohydrate is best consumed during a run? Although glucose is absorbed quickly, a mixture of sugars in dilute solutions, is preferable, especially when taken every 30 minutes or so during the run. Sports drinks such as Gatorade and/or gels are popular.

CARBOHYDRATES AFTER RUNNING

1. As we have seen earlier, glycogen is stored quickly when carbohydrates are taken within one hour of finishing a run. Even after this period and up to 24 hours, glycogen will continue to be stored but at a reduced rate.

2. So, for a quicker recovery, eat complex carbohydrates 1.0-1.5 gram/ kg of body weight, preferably 15-30 minutes after a run. You should repeat this after 2 hours.

3. If you are running a couple of times per day, recovery time is critical. If glycogen stores are grossly reduced, performance in the second run will be below par.

4. To avoid this, follow the procedure mentioned above. Drink or eat complex carbohydrates at the rate of 1.0-1.5 gram/ kg of body weight straight after the first run. Repeat 2 hours before the second run, keep refueling when needed and also just before the start of the next run.

HOW DO MUSCLES USE FOOD AS FUEL?

The muscles have two systems by which they produce energy: *the aerobic and anaerobic systems.*

As the name implies, the anaerobic system does not use oxygen in converting fuel into energy since this is a very fast process. For example, when a seasoned track athlete is running 100 metres, the only fuel needed by his fast-contracting muscles is glucose. The glucose he needs is derived from the glycogen stored in his muscles, which breaks down to supply the glucose needed to satisfy his intense energy requirement.

In contrast, when one goes for a long training run, the aerobic system is used to provide the energy required over a longer period of time, with oxygen helping to burn the fuel. *Here, the muscles are not working as intensely as in the anaerobic system and they can be active for a longer time although at a lower intensity.* A mixture of carbohydrates, protein and fat is used as fuel to supply the energy required.

Most of the distance running that joggers do involves running generally at a slow pace with occasional bouts of speed, such as in fartlek running. So, a combination of aerobic and anaerobic metabolism is involved with the energy required coming not only from carbohydrates but also from protein and fats.

RACE DISTANCE	AEROBIC USED	ANAEROBIC USED
100 meters	0%	100%
400 meters	25%	75%
5 kilometres	88%	12%
10 kilometers	97%	3%
42.2 kilometers	100%	0%

FAST-TWITCH AND SLOW-TWITCH MUSCLES

1. There are two types of muscle fibres: fast-twitch and slow-twitch.

2. Fast-twitch muscles contract very quickly, giving energy rapidly for periods ranging from 30 seconds to about 2 minutes. Thus they are used for sprinting and, as expected, they work anaerobically.

3. Slow-twitch muscles, on the other hand, contract slower but can work for a longer period of time. They use the aerobic system to give them energy for the extended periods that long, slow runs require.

According to the Canada Food Guide, you should be getting most of your carbohydrate from grains, fruits and vegetables. *About 9 servings of grains, cereal, bread, rice or pasta and 5 servings each of fruits and vegetables daily are recommended.* These will also supply you with the necessary vitamins, minerals, fibre, antioxidants and other phytochemicals. For example, grains also contain the B vitamins thiamin, riboflavin, and niacin, which are needed to convert the carbohydrate you eat into energy. Note that a serving, in the case of bread, is represented by one thin slice while a glass of orange juice is equivalent to one serving of fruit.

The energy needs of a runner can be quite high, depending on the intensity and mileage. As mentioned before, running just one kilometer can require about 65 extra calories. If you run or train for longer than that, you will require more carbohydrate for energy. Depending on the intensity and length of the run, the carbohydrate requirements may vary from 6g to 10g per kg of body weight. This is equivalent to eating about 408g to 680g of carbohydrate for a 68 kg/150 lb runner.

CARBOHYDRATES IN SOME FRUITS AND VEGETABLES

Fruit	Carbohydrate(g)	Calories
1 Banana	26	100
1 Apple	18	70
1 Strawberry	1	4
1 Orange	16	65
1 Pear	25	100
1 Peach	7	35
1 Avocado	12	227
1 Grapefruit	23	100
100g Blueberries	15	49
100g Grapes (20)	15	50

Vegetable (100g cooked)	Carbohydrate(g)	Calories
Beetroot	9	38
Broccoli	1	32
Carrot	5	32
Tomatoes	4	36
Spinach	1	23
Potatoes (boiled)	21	90
Potatoes (baked)	21	92
Sweet potatoes (baked)	20	90

Juices	Carbohydrate(g)	Calories
Orange (1 cup)	25	110
Apple (1 cup, 248g)	28	114
Grapefruit (1cup, 247g)	23	96
Tomato (1 cup, 243g)	10	41

Table 2

CARBOHYDRATES IN BREADS, CEREALS AND COOKIES

Bread - 100g Serving	Carbohydrate(g)	Calories
White	46	235
Whole grain	43	265
Whole Grain toasted (4 slices)	47	288
White toasted (6 thin slices)	65	300
Cinnamon Raisin Bagel	55	273
Croissant	27	230

Cereal - 100g Serving	Carbohydrate(g)	Calories
Oatmeal, cooked (1 cup)	60	360
Oat bran	68	375
Kellogg's Corn Flakes	82	350
Cheerios (3½ cups)	75	367
Pasta, cooked	77	365
White rice, cooked	28	119

Cookies	Carbohydrate(g)	Calories
Chocolate Chip (8)	65	454
Peanut Butter (6)	58	457
Wheat Bran Muffin	73	396

Table 3

As a rough guide, you'll get 50 grams of carbohydrate in each of the following: 4 pieces of whole-grain toast, one large bowl of breakfast cereal or porridge with milk, 1 medium baked potato, one plateful of boiled rice or pasta, two cups of orange juice or two bananas.

EARLY MORNING RUNS

Running on an empty stomach first thing in the morning is not a good idea. The glycogen stores in the liver are apt to be rather low as some of it has been used up during sleep to fuel breathing, heart beat, blood flow and other normal body functions. So, to get energy the body may start to break muscle mass in order to burn the released protein and fat. This can be avoided by eating some carbohydrate before the early morning run.

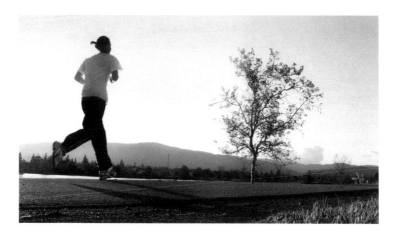

TIPS FOR INCREASING CARBOHYDRATE STORAGE
FOR MARATHON RUNNERS

Most distance training such as for marathons calls for a week of tapering off before race day. During the last week of your training, reduce the duration of your daily runs from 60 to 20 minutes for the first 4 days, followed by two days of total rest just before the race.

Since you are reducing the distance you are running during that time, you could also decrease the calorie intake from 60% to 40%

for the first 3 days of that week. For the last three days, increase your carbohydrate consumption to 70% of your daily total calories. This will allow your glycogen stores to be at their maximum.

In summary:

DAY NUMBER	RUNNING TIME	CARBO INTAKE
1	60 minutes	60%
2	40 minutes	50%
3	30 minutes	40%
4	20 minutes	70%
5	0 minute	70%
6	0 minute	70%
7	Race Day	

Table 4

For endurance events such as marathons, evidence suggests that consuming energy bars, candies, jelly gums or sports drinks about half an hour before the start may be beneficial by topping up the body's energy stores. However, one should first try these foods during training, as some runners may not be able to run well after a rise in the blood glucose level. ◆

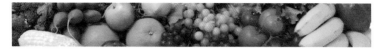

CHAPTER 3

PROTEINS

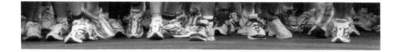

All parts of our body, including muscles, tendons, ligaments, blood, bones and skin, are made of protein, which overall constitute about 20% of the body. *Not only do proteins build the various parts of the body but they also repair them when damaged.* In fact, proteins in the body are continuously being broken down and rebuilt to renew our body parts.

Proteins are broken down during digestion into a total of twenty-two amino acids, ten of which are known as essential amino acids since they are not formed in the body due to lack of the necessary enzymes for their biosynthesis. They must, therefore, be obtained from our food. *All the amino acids are necessary in order to build up our muscles and other parts of the body.*

Foods that contain all the essential amino acids are known as complete proteins. Foods from animal sources such as meat, fish, eggs, milk and products derived from milk have complete proteins.

The ten essential amino acids are: histidine, isoleucine, leucine, lysine, methionine, phenylalanine, threonine, tryptophan, valine and arginine. Although arginine is listed as being an essential amino acid, it is required only for children but not for adults.

While animal proteins contain all the essential amino acids, proteins from vegetable sources such as dried beans, split peas and lentils may lack one or more. The only exception is soy which is also a complete protein. For example, cereals lack lysine while beans are low on methionine and cysteine. *Vegetable proteins, therefore, have to be eaten in combination with other foods for the body to be able to use the protein effectively.*

MATCHING INCOMPLETE PLANT PROTEINS

Incomplete proteins from plants can be divided into three groups:

1. Legumes: beans of all kinds, peas and lentils.
2. Grains: rice, barley, wheat and corn.
3. Nuts and seeds: walnuts, peanuts, sesame, sunflower and pumpkin seeds.

By preparing dishes containing any two of these three groups, you'll get all the essential amino acids that the body needs.

This has been known for millennia and has given rise to well-known dishes which *combine grains with legumes such as corn tortillas and beans or rice with peas or lentils.*

Dairy products such as milk, yoghurt, cheese are not only complete proteins but they also have extra amino acids that can complement those missing in grains and seeds.

Compared to sedentary people, *runners need more protein to help repair their muscles, tendons and blood vessels that get damaged during running.* A lack of protein in the diet will result in poor stamina, slower recovery from heavy training and a poor immune system. Fortunately, most of us in Canada get more protein in our regular diet than we really need.

Excessive consumption of protein could result in lowering your intake of carbohydrates. This could have a negative impact on your glycogen levels and hence your running times.
During protein metabolism, ammonia is formed and is normally excreted in the urine. However, if protein is taken in excess of

what the body requires, the large volume of ammonia formed is also released through the sweat.

PROTEIN REQUIREMENTS FOR RUNNERS

1. If you are running regularly, you'll need to eat about one gram of protein per kilogram of body weight (1.0g/kg) daily.

2. A 75 kg runner will, therefore, need around 75 grams of protein, which can be obtained from 2- 3 servings of meat, poultry, fish or eggs per day. Long distance runners may need more, 1.0-1.8g/kg.

3. A runner eating per day, one egg, a cup of dried beans, one serving of meat or fish (or 2 servings of soy) and 3 servings of low-fat milk or other dairy products will also satisfy all her protein requirements.

4. It is a good idea to include some protein with each of your meals but especially after a run.

5. Do not eat a high protein meal just before a run. Since it takes longer for the body to digest protein, it may stay in your stomach during the race and cause cramping.

Animal sources of protein usually contain appreciable amounts of saturated fats. So, if you are a meat eater, you should try and always choose leaner cuts of meat and low-fat dairy products.

PROTEIN REQUIRED PER Kg OF BODY WEIGHT						
Body weight kg or (lb)	1.4	1.5	1.6	1.7	1.8	1.9
50 (110)	70	75	80	85	90	95
59 (130)	83	89	94	100	106	112
68 (150)	95	102	109	116	122	129
77(170)	108	109	123	131	139	146

Table 5

An average runner needs around 1.2 to 1.8 g per kg of body weight. So, from the above table, a 68 kg (150 lb) runner would need a daily intake of 109 g of protein at the rate of 1.6g per kilogram of body weight.

Although most of the energy we need while running comes from carbohydrates, the body will also use proteins and fats as fuel sources in long runs when it is getting short on carbohydrates. For example, it is estimated that towards the last stage of a marathon, about 10% of the energy of marathoners come from proteins and fats.

The body cannot store large amounts of protein, so any excess protein is transformed into glucose or fat. *Consuming excessive amounts of protein also requires a higher water intake in order to degrade the amine portion of the amino acids and flush it out as ammonia in the urine and sweat.*

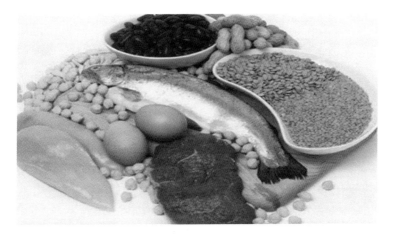

Proteins are absorbed at different rates by the body. Both slow and fast-acting amino acids are needed for repairing muscle damage that may continue for several hours after running.

So, for post-run refueling, you should eat, as soon as possible, a mixture of carbohydrate and protein in small amounts several times rather than in one big meal. For optimum result, about 0.10g of protein per kg of body weight is necessary. The average runner can get this amount of protein by eating a piece of toast with a glass of milk or chocolate milk.

We have already seen in Chapter 2 how carbohydrates help in the release of insulin. We also now know that insulin helps funnel amino acids, formed by the breakdown of proteins, into muscles after running. This explains why taking some carbohydrates and proteins straight after a tiring run will lead to less breakdown of muscle protein, resulting in less muscle soreness. Furthermore, research at McMaster University has indicated that protein synthesis is important for the muscle recovery process and that eating some protein after a run will speed up the repair.

A 2010 Dutch study, published in the American Journal of Clinical Nutrition, showed that eating protein after 30 minutes of exercise resulted in the body converting more protein into muscle than when at rest. ♦

FOOD	PROTEIN (g)
Chicken (100g)	22
Beef (85g)	24
Ham (85g)	21
Salmon (85g)	22
Turkey (85g)	21
Tuna (60g)	14
Milk (225g)	8
Cheese (28g)	7
Egg (medium)	6
Kidney Beans (½ cup)	8
Lentils (1 cup)	18
Hummus (¼ cup)	5
Almonds (28g)	6
Peanuts (½ cup)	19
Walnuts (½ cup)	10
Whole wheat bread (28g slice)	3
Pasta (1 cup)	6.5
White rice (1 cup)	2.5
Brown rice (1 cup)	6

Table 6

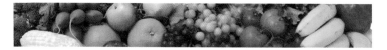

CHAPTER 4

FATS

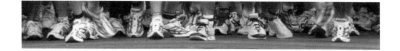

There are three main types of fats: saturated, monounsaturated and polyunsaturated.

Saturated fats are found mostly in animal-derived foods such as fatty meat, whole milk, butter, cheese, cream and lard. Saturated fats are converted into cholesterol by the liver. A diet rich in animal fats will raise the 'bad' or LDL cholesterol and increases the risk of heart disease.

Unsaturated fats exist in the monounsaturated and polyunsaturated forms. These are the 'good' fats as they tend to raise levels of the 'good' or HDL cholesterol and lower the 'bad' or LDL cholesterol. Consumption of these fats lowers the risk of heart disease and offers a whole host of other health benefits.

Monounsaturated fats are found in olive oil, canola oil and peanut oil. Polyunsaturated oils are also found in vegetable oils such as those derived from soybeans and safflower.

Omega-3 fats are a special class of polyunsaturated fats which are found in nut oils, flaxseed, walnut, canola and especially fish oils. Numerous studies have shown that a diet rich in omega-3 fats reduces the risk of heart disease.

So, fats especially the good ones, should be an essential part of our diet. Fats provide more than twice the calories of either carbohydrates or proteins. In addition to providing calories for the runner, fats are also necessary for the formation of important hormones such as the sex hormones. They are involved as well in the absorption of many vitamins such as the fat-soluble vitamins A and E. Since the fat that we eat can eventually be stored as body fat, we have to limit our consumption to mostly low-fat foods, not exceeding about 20% of total calories.

GOOD FATS

1. Monounsaturated, polyunsaturated and omega-3 fats are all good fats.

2. The good fats lower the 'bad' LDL-cholesterol and raise the 'good' HDL-cholesterol.

3. An increase in LDL-cholesterol increases your risk of heart disease and stroke.

4. Monounsaturated fats are found in vegetable and nut oils such as olive, canola, avocado and almond.

5. Dietary polyunsaturated fats are largely made up of two groups, the omega-6 and omega-3 fats.

6. Omega-6 fats are found in corn, soybean, sesame and safflower oils.

7. Omega-3 fats are found in fish oils, nuts, flaxseed and soy.

8. Studies have shown that a diet high in omega-3 fats is especially helpful in keeping total cholesterol low and reducing the risk of coronary artery disease.

Runners should be aware that although fats are a good source of fuel, it takes a long time to digest them. Although this is a disadvantage in the short term, it nevertheless makes us feel full and so prevents us from suffering pangs of hunger during a long run.

As runners increase their fitness levels, they develop the ability to burn more fat while running at higher intensities. In so doing, depletion of glycogen levels is delayed.

BAD FATS
1. Saturated fats and trans fats are 'bad' fats.
2. Even though they are 'bad' fats, saturated fats are needed by the body. However, we should be careful not to get more than about 10% of our total calories from saturated fats since the liver uses saturated fats to make cholesterol, mostly LDL-cholesterol.
3. A high LDL-cholesterol could increase the risk of heart disease.
4. Saturated fats are found mostly in foods from animal sources such as whole milk, butter, cheese, cream and fatty meat. Tropical oils such as coconut and palm oils are also high in saturated fats.
5. Trans fats are formed when mono and polyunsaturated fats from plant-derived oils are hydrogenated to form margarine. Some trans fats occur naturally in very small quantities in milk and meat.
6. Trans fats are worse for you than saturated fats since they not only 'raise' the 'bad' LDL-cholesterol but also lower the 'good' HDL-cholesterol. Trans fats are found in hard margarine, shortening, fast food fries, chips, cookies, and other packaged foods.

So, do your heart a lot of good by limiting your consumption of red meat and full-fat milk products as well as replacing the 'bad' fats especially the trans fats by 'good' ones such as omega-3 fats from oily fish.

Fats are also important as a source of energy especially for prolonged athletic activities such as marathon running. When glycogen is in short supply in the late stages of a marathon, the body switches to burning fat for energy. The better trained a runner is, the more fat he'll be able to burn while still running at moderate intensity.

USING FATS AS A SOURCE OF ENERGY

1. At 9 calories per gram, fats provide more than twice the calories that carbohydrate or protein supply, about 4 calories per gram.

2. Since fats take much longer than carbohydrate or protein to digest, they should not be eaten less than about 4 hours before a run otherwise stomach distress may occur.

3. By the same token, energy from fats is not readily available during a run. In order to be used as fuel, fats require oxygen to be present and so can only be used in aerobic workouts. This usually occurs in running of moderate intensity lasting around 2-3 hours or more.

4. It has been found that in long-distance running, seasoned and highly trained runners can use more fat as fuel and at a higher intensity than a novice. It is perhaps not surprising to find that slow-twitch muscles have more enzymes that help burn fat than their fast-twitch counterparts.

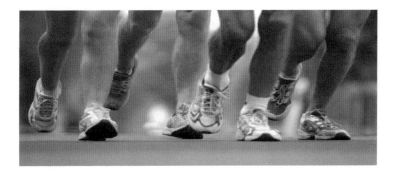

DAILY FAT REQUIREMENTS FOR RUNNERS

- In order to calculate the runner's fat requirements, one has to first add together the calories derived from carbohydrate and protein.
- Then this is subtracted from the total daily calories to yield the calories from fat.
- Since a gram of fat gives off 9 calories, the equivalent grams of fat can be calculated.

SAMPLE CALCULATION FOR THE DAILY FAT REQUIREMENT OF A 68kg (150lb) RUNNER

Carbohydrate required at 6g per kg of body weight = **408g** *(sourced from Table 4)*
Protein required at 1.6g per kg of body weight = **109g** *(sourced from Table 5)*
Total grams of carbohydrate + protein = 408g + 109g = **517g**

Since one gram of carbohydrate or protein supplies 4 calories, the equivalent calories for carbohydrate and protein would be:

517g x 4 = 2068 calories

Total daily calories for the female running 10 km = **2310 calories** (from BMR calculation in Chapter 8) + 650 calories (10 X 65 per km) = 2960 calories

Calories from fat = 2960 - 2068 = 892 calories

Since 1 gram of fat gives off 9 calories, therefore the equivalent grams of fat is equal to 892g/9 = **99.1g**

So, the daily intake should be:

carbohydrate = **408g**
protein = **109g**
fat = **99g**

MEAL	CARBS	PROTEIN	FATS
Breakfast	100	30	20
Snack before run	25	0	0
Gatorade during run	15	0	0
Recovery snack	60	20	10
Lunch	100	25	33
Dinner	108	34	36
Total	408	109	99

Total calories is equal to: [(408g + 109g) x 4 calories/gram] + (99g x 9 calories/gram) = **2959 calories**

You can then distribute the total nutrients among all your meals throughout the day, taking into consideration the time of your run. For example, if you are running at 10:00am, you would arrange to have breakfast at 7.00-8.00am, a pre-run snack at 9:30–9:45am, refueling with a sports drink during the run, a recovery snack just less than one hour after your run, lunch at 1:30–2:00pm and dinner at 6:00–7:00pm. ♦

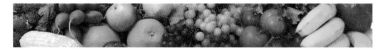

CHAPTER 5

VITAMINS

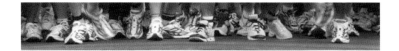

Vitamins as well as minerals are micronutrients necessary for metabolic processes which are involved in energy production from the carbohydrates, protein and fat that we eat.

If you are eating enough calories and following a varied diet with an adequate intake of fresh fruits and vegetables, you would be getting all of the necessary micronutrients.

There is no need to rely on multivitamin supplements, except perhaps for elite runners who follow a heavy training schedule or those following a vegan diet.

Strict vegetarians, especially those who eschew milk and milk products, may be deficient in vitamin B12. In the circumstances, a vitamin B12 supplement may be considered.

Although all the vitamins are essential for a healthy body, *the following vitamins are especially important for runners: vitamin B complex, vitamins C, D, E and K.* Why are these vitamins important? And why are B-vitamins so important for runners?

IMPORTANCE OF B-VITAMINS FOR RUNNERS

1. Vitamin B1 or thiamine is important for carbohydrate metabolism and energy production. Beef, beans, peas, rice and whole grains are good sources of the vitamin.

2. Vitamin B2, or riboflavin helps in the conversion of carbohydrates and fats into energy for the muscles. It is found in milk and milk products, whole grains, cereals and bread.

3. Vitamin B3 or niacin is involved in the synthesis of glycogen and releasing energy from the metabolism of carbohydrate, protein and fat. Running long distances regularly may require more niacin. It is found in whole grains, beans, meat and fish.

4. Vitamin B6 or pyridoxine is also involved in energy production. It also helps in releasing iron from the diet which in turn makes more hemoglobin. This, of course, provides more oxygen for the muscles. It works in conjunction with vitamin B2 and magnesium. Good sources of vitamin B6 are bananas, avocadoes, carrots, vegetables, rice, whole wheat flour, bran, wheat germ, beans, salmon and tuna. Canned and frozen foods contain less of the vitamin compared to the fresh ones.

5. Vitamin B12 is vital for the formation of red blood cells and nerve fibres. It is found in red meat, fish, eggs, milk and milk products. Vegans may need a B12 supplement as the non-heme iron found in vegetable and non-meat sources are not readily absorbed by the body. Aging runners also may need extra vitamin B12 because of reduced absorption by the stomach.

6. In addition to vitamin B12, other nutrients needed for the synthesis of red blood cells are vitamin B6, folic acid, vitamin C, vitamin E, iron and zinc.

VITAMIN B COMPLEX

Niacin, thiamine and riboflavin are the B vitamins necessary for the metabolism of carbohydrate, protein and fat. However, *there is no evidence that taking extra doses from supplements will make you more energetic.*

The B vitamins are water-soluble and any excess is excreted in the urine. The tiny amounts that are used up should be replaced daily. About a third of seniors have been found to lack adequate stomach acid, so they may not be able to extract enough vitamin B12 from their food. Since B vitamins are involved in energy metabolism and also in processing alcohol, boozing may make you feel out of sorts. Furthermore, alcohol causes dehydration which can add to the discomfort while running.

VITAMIN C

It is a water-soluble antioxidant which increases energy production and also helps in iron absorption. About 90 mg is needed daily for men and 75 mg for women. However, if you suffer from hemochromatosis, a disease caused by the body absorbing and storing too much iron, you have to avoid getting too much of the vitamin. *If you eat lots of fruits and vegetables, you will get all the vitamin C that you need.* People with such a diet have been found to have lower risks of certain cancers and heart disease. However, clinical trials with vitamin C pills did not show such protection. This is probably due to the fact that unlike fruits and vegetables, vitamin C pills lack fibre and other phytochemicals. Vitamin C helps build a good immunity. It is involved in the synthesis of collagen which is necessary for making connective tissue and bone. Runners also need it to help blisters and other running wounds heal. It is found in oranges, bell peppers, melons, spinach and berries.

VITAMIN E

A fat-soluble antioxidant which is thought to protect body tissues such as muscles against damage by free radicals released during running. Vitamin E is also needed for the formation of red blood cells and for helping the body use vitamin K. It is found in nuts, seeds, corn, avocadoes, vegetable oils and wheat germ. Margarine and other products made from vegetable oils also contain vitamin E. Although at low levels, vitamin E protects the heart, at much higher levels (greater than 400 IU per day), it could increase your risk of dying, according to the American Heart Association.

VITAMIN K

It is a fat-soluble vitamin which is found as phylloquinone in plants and as menaquinones when synthesized by intestinal bacteria. It is needed for good coagulation of blood and for bone health. Vitamin K activates proteins which cause the blood to clot at the site of a cut. It is also essential for the role of calcium in bone building. It is found in green, leafy vegetables such as spinach, chard and kale as well as members of the cruciferous vegetables such as broccoli and cabbage. It is also found in soybeans, milk and milk products.

VITAMIN D

The recommended dose for the fat-soluble vitamin D is 1000 IU daily. *If you regularly eat vitamin D-rich foods such as fatty fish, fortified dairy products and eggs, you probably are getting enough vitamin D and may not need supplements. It is also important to get some sun exposure, especially around noon, since the vitamin is formed by the action of sunshine on the skin.* Vitamin D is necessary for the absorption of calcium and the maintenance of bone health. It, therefore, reduces the risk of bone fractures. It has also been found to reduce muscle weakness, especially in the elderly. More recently, vitamin D has been found to reduce the risk of many diseases including cancer, diabetes, heart disease and several immune diseases.

You can get all the vitamins you need from a healthy diet consisting of fresh fruits, vegetables, milk, cheese, yogurt and other milk products, whole wheat products, eggs, meat and fish.

Vitamins are essential for good health which, in turn, is a pre-requisite for good running. There is no need to take multivitamin supplements if you are following a healthy diet. ♦

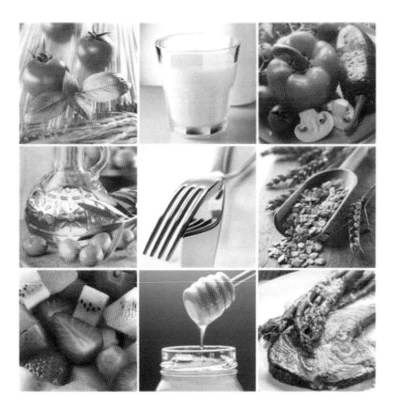

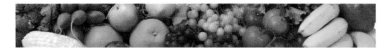

CHAPTER 6

MINERALS

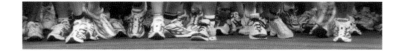

Intense running affects the level of most minerals in the body and in particular, sodium, potassium, iron and calcium.

Your performance will suffer if these minerals are not at their optimum levels. In most cases a supplement is not necessary since a nutrient-rich diet will supply enough vitamins and minerals for even the advanced runner. Furthermore, there is no evidence to suggest that taking vitamin supplements to boost vitamin levels improves our running performance. Let's see how these minerals are involved in running:

IRON

As we have seen previously, *iron is needed for making red blood cells which carry oxygen to the muscles and organs.* Heme-iron is found in red meat, dark chicken or turkey meat, eggs and seafood. Non-heme iron comes from vegetable sources such as nuts, spinach and other green vegetables. Heme-iron is more easily absorbed than non-heme iron but the absorption of both types of iron can be increased by the presence of acids, such as vitamin C or citric acid from lemon juice.

The tannins present in tea or coffee will reduce the amount of iron absorbed at mealtimes if they are drunk during meals. So, always drink these beverages in between your meals.

Most runners will not suffer from iron deficiency unless they are strict vegetarians or vegans. Older runners with reduced stomach acid, women with heavy periods and female runners who train a lot also may lack iron. Some of these young women may also have a high incidence of amenorrhea, which is a lack of menstrual bleeding. This condition prevents the iron level from falling further.

Low iron stores, which can be determined by a ferritin test, will make runners feel weak and tired since the blood will no longer be able to carry oxygen adequately to the muscles.

Men should get around 8 mg of iron per day and women need more, about 20 mg. Be wary of taking an excess of iron from supplements since it could reduce the absorption of zinc.

CALCIUM

Calcium is needed for good muscle function and to build strong bones for reducing the risk of osteoporosis and stress fractures. It helps control blood pressure and is involved in muscle contraction. *Vitamin D is needed for its absorption.* Consuming black coffee could increase excretion of calcium but this can be avoided by adding some milk to it.

Good sources of calcium include dairy products, seafood, sardines, tofu, oranges, nuts, beans and dark vegetables. You should aim for around 1,000 mg of calcium per day. Calcium deficiency is more common in women than men.

Although running will help women build stronger bones, they could still lose bone mass if they suffer from amenorrhea.

In addition to having low iron levels, these women will also be lacking estrogen, a hormone that helps in maintaining bone mass. This can be remedied by increasing consumption of calcium-containing foods or taking a supplement containing calcium and vitamin D.

POTASSIUM

Together with sodium and chloride ions, potassium is involved in the regulation of fluid balance and in controlling how muscles and nerves act. It also helps in transporting glucose to muscles.

Potassium is found in avocadoes, potatoes, yoghurt, beans, spinach, bananas, oranges, grapefruit, carrots, broccoli and milk.

Most people including runners tend to consume too much sodium but not enough potassium. So make sure that your diet contains lots of vegetables, fruits and dairy products to increase your level of potassium.

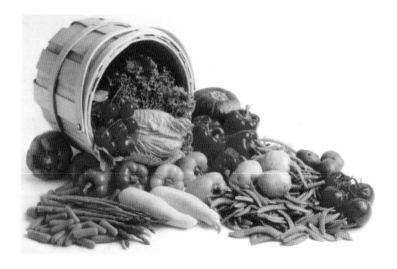

SODIUM

As running intensity increases, sweating occurs and small amounts of electrolytes including sodium are lost. Although a balanced diet will replace sodium, long distance runners and those running for more than 90 minutes, should consume additional sodium during their runs by drinking a sports drink such as Gatorade. *However, care has to be taken in order not to drink excessive amounts of water, which could dangerously lower the sodium levels.* Sodium is found in salt, salty snacks and canned soups.

Most runners will consume higher levels of sodium since it is found in all kinds of prepared foods. So, to cut back on sodium, eat more food that you have prepared yourself.

MAGNESIUM

As magnesium is responsible for the level of calcium in tissues, *an inadequate amount may result in muscle cramps.* By improving calcium absorption, it also strengthens bones. The recommended daily intake is 320 mg for women and 420mg for men.

It is found in halibut, almonds, peanuts, spinach, potato, whole grains, avocado, green and leafy vegetables, beans and peas. You could try magnesium supplements if your diet is low in the mineral and you do not suffer from kidney disease.

ZINC

Zinc is important for building a strong immune system and for the proper functioning of a multitude of enzymes in the body.

These are involved, for example, in the formation of DNA, RNA, proteins and collagen.

After intense running, there is an appreciable loss of zinc. So, foods rich in zinc such as lentils, nuts, shrimps, oysters and other seafood, turkey, beef and broccoli should be consumed regularly by long-distance runners.

CHROMIUM

Insulin needs chromium in order to help the body use glucose, amino acids and fats. Chromium is found in brewer's yeast, black pepper, liver and whole grains.

COPPER

Copper, together with iron, is a trace element which is involved in oxygen metabolism as a result of the mediation of several enzymes. It plays a role in keeping our bones healthy. It is found in meat, beans, whole grains, potatoes, dried fruits, shellfish and liver.

ANTIOXIDANTS

Free radicals such as reactive oxygen species are formed during normal body processes but more are generated during exercise, including running. We are also exposed to free radicals as a result of environmental factors such air pollution, UV radiation from the sun and smoke.

Free radicals increase damage to cells and, more importantly, damage DNA and so increase the risk of diseases such as cancer and heart disease.

The large volumes of oxygen that we breathe in while running generate more free radicals, which increase the oxidative stress on our cells. They get damaged in the process resulting in sore muscles, fatigue and increased inflammation.

Antioxidants are compounds that reduce oxidative stress in the body and so protect cells against damage caused by free radicals. In short, they mop up the damaging free radicals.

Studies done over the last 30 years have shown many benefits of antioxidants in the diet, including a reduction in muscle damage and improved performance, as long as we consume enough of them.

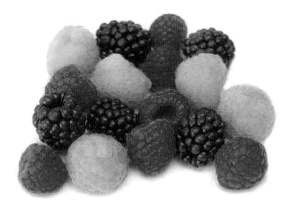

A recent paper in the 'Journal of the International Society of Sports Nutrition' gave some hope to sprinters over 50 trying to regain the running times they had in the previous 5-10 years. It found that taking a mixture of antioxidants together with the amino acid, arginine, increased anaerobic threshold as a result of reduction of lactic acid accumulation in the blood, especially in the over 50's. Surprisingly perhaps, no change in the VO2 max was observed. (VO2 max. is the maximum volume of oxygen, per kg of body weight, one can breathe in while exercising at one's maximum. The fitter you are, the higher your VO2 max. will be).

Common antioxidants include vitamins such as vitamins A, C and E and minerals such as selenium, copper and manganese.

In addition to providing many vitamins and minerals, fruits and vegetables, especially brightly coloured ones, are loaded with different types of antioxidants and other phytochemicals. Some of these phytochemicals include carotenoids, flavonoids, isothiocyanates, phenols and sulfides. *They appear to be more effective when they work in synergy with one another, as when found in fresh fruits and vegetables.*

With some rare exceptions, most studies of antioxidant *supplements*, including an analysis of 67 trials involving 230,000 patients, do not show any beneficial effect on mortality. In fact, a study of the antioxidant vitamins A, E and beta-carotene in *supplements* actually slightly increased the risk of death!

Eating the whole fruit is better for you than drinking the corresponding juice since it will also supply much needed fibre and other nutrients.

According to the Canada Food Guide, an adult should consume 3 to 5 servings of fruit every day. Brightly coloured fruits such as berries, oranges, apples, peaches, cherries, kiwis, mangoes, pineapple, melons and pomegranate are high in antioxidants.

Antioxidants are also found in dark chocolate, nuts, spices, herbs, whole grains and vegetables such as spinach, tomatoes, carrots, peppers, onions, garlic, eggplants, cabbages, broccoli, kale and cauliflower.

Other important sources of antioxidants in the diet include cocoa, tea and coffee.

Many studies have purported to show that the antioxidants in coffee are related to caffeine and chlorogenic acids which are found in green, unroasted coffee beans. However, scientists at the University of British Columbia writing in 'Food Research International' found that most of these acids are destroyed during the roasting process. They claimed that a new class of antioxidants, known as Maillard reaction products, is formed during roasting of the beans. ♦

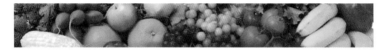

CHAPTER 7

HYDRATION

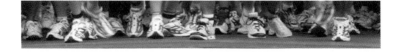

Good hydration for runners is necessary before, during and after running. Water makes up about half of our body's weight. *When we run, the body generates heat and we sweat in order to keep us cool.* When it's humid, sweat evaporates less and it becomes harder to cool the body. So, it gets more difficult for you to work at your usual intensity.

When we lose water through sweat, we have to drink more in order to keep the body's temperature down, especially during long runs. Also, metabolic processes require water, so to keep running efficiently the water lost through sweat has to be replaced.

Sweat formation decreases when one becomes dehydrated. The blood volume diminishes and the blood becomes thicker. It then gets harder for the heart to pump blood to your muscles and also to get rid of excess heat. When this happens, the body's temperature can become so high that heatstroke could result.

One should drink even before becoming thirsty since the body does not have a good thirst mechanism. If you wait to drink until you get thirsty, you may already be somewhat dehydrated. As water is needed to dilute waste products before they are excreted, a lack of water will reduce urine flow and turn it dark and cloudy. Other signs of dehydration while running include nausea, chills and dizziness.

How much one needs to drink depends on the day's temperature, humidity and how hard the run is. If you run fast and for a long time, you'll sweat more and have a greater need to drink fluid.

Running for 1 hour or less needs only plain water for rehydration. For longer runs, the electrolytes that you lose, such as sodium, chloride and potassium, have to be replaced by taking Gatorade or Powerade and other sports drinks or sports gels.

Don't forget to drink half a cup of water with the gel so as to get the correct dilution for quick absorption. This will ensure that you have energy left for the end of the run. In general, during a run, a well hydrated runner lasts longer (up to 20%) than one who is not adequately hydrated. However, do not overindulge since sports drinks such as Gatorade have lots of calories, about 240 per liter.

The average loss of electrolytes per liter of sweat are as follows: sodium, 1150mg; potassium, 250 mg; calcium, 28 mg ; magnesium, 50 mg and chloride, 1480 mg. (Adapted from Andrew Hamilton, Peak Performance Issue 212).

Loss of water and electrolytes during long runs can cause muscle cramps. However, be careful about taking pain medications just before or during a run. Pain relievers such as Advil and aspirin, but not Tylenol, can affect blood flow to the kidneys and the retention of sodium. Drinking coffee or tea may be counterproductive since they'll increase urination in the short term. So, you may need to drink even more to replace the water lost.

The most effective energy gels should ideally contain not just carbohydrate and minerals but some protein too. Researchers at James Madison University have recently found that when a sports drink has a carbohydrate to protein ratio of 4:1, endurance was increased by 15% and muscle damage was also reduced.

Some studies have shown that drinking a sports drink while running is also good for the immune system, which is depressed for several hours after a prolonged bout of exercise.

The trend in sports drinks such as Gatorade (PepsiCo), Powerade (Coca-Cola) and Lucozade (Glaxo Smith Kline) is to nutritionally target the different stages of exercising and running: pre-run, during run and post-run.

A pre-run sports drink will ideally contain carbohydrates, sodium and potassium, together with some B-vitamins which are involved in releasing energy such as B3, B5 and B6. The sports drink to take during runs contains carbohydrates and electrolytes such as sodium and potassium while the post-run drink contains the same nutrients plus some protein to help muscles heal.

HYDRATION BEFORE RUNNING

1. The amount of fluid to drink depends on the temperature and humidity. If it's hot, you'll need to drink more than if it's a cool day.

2. Do not gulp down large volumes of fluids in one go, rather drink small amounts frequently throughout the day.

3. Drink a couple of cups of cool water 1-2 hours before your run.

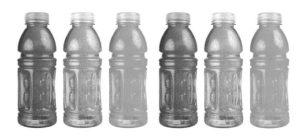

HYDRATION WHILE RUNNING

1. You need to drink some water or sports drink every 20-30 minutes during a run, especially if it is hot and you perspire a lot.

2. At water stations, walk in order to be able to drink more and avoid gulping it down.

3. However, don't drink excessive amounts of water while running as this could reduce the sodium level of your blood to such dangerous low levels, 130 mmol/L or less, as to cause hyponatremia.

4. Since sports drinks have a lower sodium concentration than the blood, they too can cause hyponatremia if drunk to excess.

HYDRATION AFTER RUNNING

1. After a run, you need to rehydrate.

2. Replace the weight lost during a run by consuming water until you have reached your pre-run weight.

3. Drinking water after a run also helps to clean out the body's waste products.

4. Clear, pale yellow urine indicates that rehydration is complete.

5. Avoid beer for hydration after running as alcohol is a diuretic.

WATER LOSS AND SWEAT RATE CALCULATION

Weigh yourself before a run, preferably with no clothes on. After your run, don't go to the bathroom until you have dried yourself and taken your weight again as before. The difference is the weight of sweat you have lost. Repeat for several days and take the average.

Average weight lost in kilograms x 1000 = number of ml of sweat lost (since 1 kg=1000g and the density of water is 1.00g/ml)

If you are used to drinking a certain volume of fluid during your run, add that volume to the number of ml of sweat lost to get your total sweat lost.

Divide this amount by the length of time of the run in hours and you'll get your hourly sweat rate. To rehydrate, divide your hourly sweat rate by 4 and take that amount of fluid every 15 minutes (60 minutes/4).

Drink water until your weight is as it was before your run and your urine is clear.

Weight of runner before the race = **74.5 kg**

Weight of runner after the race = **73.9 kg**

Weight lost as sweat = **74.5 - 73.9 = 0.6 kg**

Volume of sweat lost = **0.6 kg x 1000g/kg x 1.00ml/g = 600 ml**

Volume of water consumed during the 1.2 hr run = **300 ml**

Total volume of sweat lost
+ volume drunk = **600 ml + 300 ml = 900 ml**

Rate of sweat lost per hour = **900 ml/1.2 hr = 75 ml per hour**

To replace the fluid lost, the runner has to drink **75 ml in one hour.**

This is equivalent to drinking **75 m l/4 = 18.75 ml** or about **19 ml** every **15 minutes.**

DRINKING TOO MUCH FLUID CAN
IMPAIR PERFORMANCE

Despite what has been said earlier in this chapter about hydration, be wary about overdrinking during a race. Well-known sports medicine researcher, Professor Timothy Noakes of Cape Town University, has recently shown that of the 643 marathoners who completed the 2009 Mont Saint Michel Marathon, *those who drank the most fluids to make up for their sweat loss were the slowest.* Runners losing over 3% of their body weight were the fastest, finishing under 3 hours. Those who finished in 3 to 4 hours lost on average 2.5% of their body weight. These losses in body weight were unaffected by gender or age. So, moderation is as always the key!

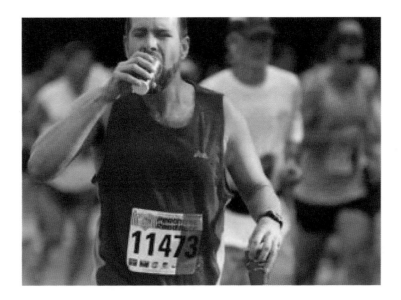

PHYSICAL SYMPTOMS RESULTING FROM FLUID LOSS

% BW Loss	Weight Loss / 67kg Man	Symptoms
1%	0.67 kg/1.50 lb	Thirsty, slower run
2%	1.34 kg/3.0 lb	Thirstier, can't eat
3%	2.0 kg/4.5 lb	Dry mouth, less urine
4%	2.7 kg/6.0 lb	Speed slower by 30 %
5%	3.4 kg/7.5 lb	Heat exhaustion

Table 7 *(International Journal of Sports Medicine, volume 15(3), pp. 122 -125, 1994)*

With more than 5% of body weight lost as sweat, the body temperature goes up drastically, breathing becomes more laboured and the runner eventually collapses. ♦

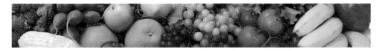

CHAPTER 8
ERGOGENIC OR PERFORMANCE ENHANCING COMPOUNDS

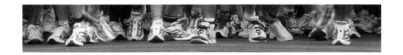

Most runners would no doubt like to have an edge on the competition and sometimes training may not be enough for the very ambitious ones. This is why the sports nutrition market is now worth $5 billion globally! However, there is much hype about many of these compounds *while their scientific validity is often lacking.*

CAFFEINE

Caffeine is a central nervous system stimulant and could improve racing times when taken in doses lower than and up to 3 mg per kg of body weight.

So, a 68 kg (150 pound) runner could consume about 205 mg of caffeine although improvement in performance shows up before this level is reached. *This amount of caffeine is found in about 2 cups (500ml) of home made, filtered coffee (150-250 mg).* Drunk about 1-2 hours before a race, it could shave off a few precious seconds from your time.

There are many studies which show that caffeine as a stimulant helps some runners improve their times in long-distance runs by up to 10%. However, runners vary in their response to caffeine, with those who do not consume coffee regularly showing the best results. The effect is negligible in high-intensity runs such as sprinting events of half an hour or less. It should be noted that *caffeine is a banned drug at the Olympics, if caffeine concentration is found to be more than 15 micrograms per milliliter of urine.*

Caffeine is not only a diuretic but it could also upset the stomach, especially if one is not used to it. However, the diuretic effect lasts only a few hours after coffee intake. In fact, a study published in the International Journal of Sports Nutrition in 2005 showed that there is no difference in the urine volume at the end of a 24-hour period whether the subjects drink one cup of coffee, several cups, no coffee at all or just plain water.

Caffeine in doses larger than 300 mg may in fact be detrimental to your racing times. Furthermore, it could cause heart beat anomalies, increase jitteriness and cause diarrhea with possible dehydration as a consequence.

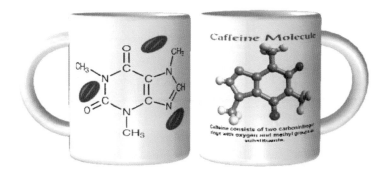

CREATINE

Creatine, a compound found in meat and fish, is effective in increasing the muscular strength, power and lean body mass of athletes. According to a 2005 review by the University of Oklahoma scientists in 'Sports Medicine', *creatine does not increase stamina in long-distance runners but improves the performance of sprinters and other short distance runners.* Creatine has some disadvantages such as slowing down healing and increasing the risk of hamstring strains.

COENZYME Q10

Coenzyme Q10 is found in the mitochondria, also known as the power house of cells. It plays an important role in the production of energy and in endurance. Around your mid-twenties, the level of coenzyme Q10 diminishes and supplementation may improve running performances. Research carried out in Japan and published in a 2008 issue of 'Nutrition' has shown that supplementation with 300 mg of coenzyme Q10 for 8 days reduced fatigue and shortened recovery time after exercise.

BEETROOT (BEETS)

Research, carried out by Professor A. Jones at Exeter University's School of Sport and Health Science, and published in the Journal of Applied Physiology in 2009, has shown that *drinking organic beetroot juice, a rich source of nitrate, can increase stamina and allow you to exercise for 15% longer than usual.*

How does it work? Drinking beetroot juice doubled the nitrate level in blood. The nitrate is converted to nitric oxide, which reduces the amount of oxygen that muscles need while exercising. So, muscles work more efficiently with less oxygen. As a result, both low and high-intensity running become less exhausting.

Boiled or pickled beetroot should also be effective although one might expect the nitrate level to be somewhat reduced.

Other sources of inorganic nitrates include green vegetables.

MILK AND CHOCOLATE MILK

There is strong evidence to show that cow's milk can be an effective drink for the recovery stage after a long run.

Research carried out at Loughborough University's School of Sports and Exercise Sciences and published in the 'British Journal of Nutrition' in 2007 showed that skimmed milk could be better for rehydration than water or Powerade.

A 2009 study from James Madison University and published in Medicine and Science in Sports and Exercise showed that compared with sports drinks having similar calories, *low fat chocolate milk works better for post run refueling since it boosts not only glycogen levels but also muscle repair.*

An enzyme showing muscle damage, creatine kinase, was found to be lower when chocolate milk is drunk soon after exercise. It is thought that the good quality protein found in milk helps in the repair of damaged muscles.

Milk also provides fluid and minerals such as potassium, calcium and magnesium to replace the amounts lost in sweat.

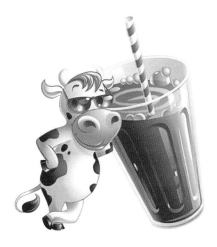

L-CARNITINE

L-Carnitine is found naturally in the body and is used for converting fat to energy.

A 2010 paper in the Journal of Physiology from researchers at the University of Nottingham Medical School found that supplementation with L-carnitine and carbohydrates for six months increased the L-carnitine level in muscles and resulted in an 11% improvement in athletic performance.

Both high and low-intensity exercises were positively affected as a result of a decrease in anaerobic energy production, the use of less muscle glycogen and a decrease in accumulation of lactic acid in the muscles.

FOLIC ACID

A 2011 paper in the 'Clinical Journal of Sports Medicine' from the Medical College of Wisconsin indicates that folic acid may improve heart health and running times for young female runners suffering from amenorrhea.

The study was done on women 18-35 who had been running a minimum of 32 km per week for a year. *Half of these women were found to be suffering from amenorrhea and also had reduced dilation in their blood vessels.* After supplementation with 10 mg of folic acid for a month, there was increased dilation in the arteries and more blood flow to the heart. The resulting increase in oxygen uptake could positively affect running performance. ♦

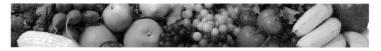

CHAPTER 9
NUTRITIONAL REQUIREMENTS
AND CALORIES

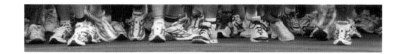

The nutritional requirements for a runner depend upon the weight, the time taken for the run and the running intensity. You can usually judge the intensity at which you are running using your 'perceived exertion rate'. This is simply your own estimation of how hard you think you are running. On a scale of 1 to 10, 1-4 is classified as low intensity, 5-7 medium intensity and 8-10 hard. For a trained runner, running at medium intensity usually means a rate of about 5 to 7 minutes per kilometre. Runners can estimate their nutritional requirements using Table 8 below.

APPROXIMATE NUTRIENT
REQUIREMENTS FOR RUNNERS

grams/kilograms

	Carbs	Protein	Fats
Low intensity for < 1 hour	5	1	0.75
Medium intensity > 1 hour	8	1.4	1.5
High intensity, long distance	10	1.8	2

Table 8

GRAMS OF NUTRIENTS NEEDED
FOR A 68 kg/150 LB RUNNER

grams

	Carbs	Protein	Fats
Low intensity for < 1 hour	340	68	51
Medium intensity > 1 hour	544	95	102
High intensity, long distance	680	122	136

Table 9

ALTERNATE ENERGY CALCULATIONS
USING CALORIES

1) The first step is to estimate the Basal Metabolic Rate (BMR), that is the number of calories the body needs for its daily activity such as to breathe, to circulate blood, to process food and in general, to perform all its vital functions, excluding any physical exercise. This can be calculated using the Harris-Benedict equation, which factors in your age, weight, height and gender. However, a simpler but less accurate way of estimating the approximate BMR is by multiplying the weight in pounds by 10 (or weight in kilograms x 22) for a woman and by 11 (weight in kilograms x 24) for a man. For example, if a female runner weighs 154 pounds (70 kg), her BMR = 154 x 10 = 1540 calories.

2) Next the runner has to determine if her lifestyle is sedentary, active or very active in order to calculate the total calories needed for the body's daily activity plus any exercise she is doing:

   a. For light running (1-3 days per week), multiply the above BMR value by 1.375

63

b. For moderate running (3-5 days a week), multiply the BMR value by 1.5

c. For heavy running (6-7 days a week), multiply the BMR by 1.7

d. For extremely hard running morning and evening, multiply BMR by 1.9

So, if the above female runs 4 days per week, her calorie expenditure would be : BMR X 1.5 = 1540 X 1.5= 2310 calories. This is only *an approximate value since her exact running distance and intensity has not been taken into account.* Obviously, she'll need more calories if she runs a 6 minute mile as opposed to a 12 minute mile for each of the four days.

As a rough guide, female and male runners require between 2000 and 2500 calories per day, to which the calories spent on running for that day has to be added.

This would be roughly 65 calories per kilometer. For the above female running 10 km a day, approximate total calories needed = 2310 calories + (10 km x 65 calories per km) = 2960 calories.

To get a more accurate result, the time taken for the run has to be factored in, by using metabolic equivalents as shown next.

A MORE ACCURATE CALCULATION FOR ENERGY NEEDS USING METABOLIC EQUIVALENTS

First we calculate the energy required just for daily living, without any running included. Then we add it to the calories used during running, by using metabolic equivalents, to get the total # of calories needed per day.

Metabolic equivalents are multiple numbers of the metabolic rate at rest, which is assumed to be 1 calorie per hour per kg of body weight. The following daily activity values are used:

Sedentary work = 1.2
Active lifestyle (not including exercise) = 1.3
Very heavy work activity = 1.5

METABOLIC EQUIVALENTS FOR
VARIOUS RUNNING SPEEDS

Running speed	Metabolic equivalent
8 km per hr = 7.5 min per km (5 mph)	8
10.8 km per hr = 5.55 min per km (6.7 mph)	11
12.1 km per hr = 4.96 min per km (7.5 mph)	12.5
16 km per hr = 3.75 min per km (10 mph)	16

Sample calculation:

a) For a 154 lb (70 kg) female runner, BMR = 154 lb x 10 = 1540 calories

b) No. of calories needed for daily living, excluding running = BMR x 1.3 for an active lifestyle. For a 70 kg (154 lb) female runner, this equals to 1540 cals x 1.3 = 2002 cal

c) If the female is running at 10.8 km/hr for 1.5 hours, from the above table, the metabolic equivalent = 11,
# of calories burnt = 70 kg x 11 x 1.5 hr = 1155 calories

d) Since the runner is running for 1.5 hr per day, one has to subtract her resting metabolic rate for 1.5 hour from her total daily living calories, 1155 calories – (70 kg x 1.5 hr) = 1155 – 105 = 1050 calories

e) Total # of calories the runner needs per day = calories needed for daily living + calories for running = 2002 cals + 1050 cals = 3052 calories

This value is thought to be a more accurate calorie requirement for the runner than the 2960 calories obtained in the previous section.

By performing a similar calculation using your own data, you can determine the total daily calories that you need in order to optimize your training and performance. ♦

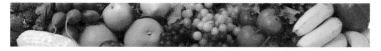

CHAPTER 10
TYPE AND TIMING OF NUTRIENTS

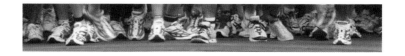

Knowing how much nutrient to eat (see Chapter 9) is not enough. We also need to know what type of nutrients to eat and when to do so.

Generally, the closer you are to starting your run, the more carbohydrate you should be consuming compared to protein and fat.

For example, about 15 minutes before your run, take about 25 grams of simple carbohydrate or about 100 calories. About 1 hour or more before the run, you can eat about 50 g of carbohydrate or 200 calories, including small amounts of protein and fat. If you are eating breakfast 2 to 3 hours before a run, you can consume about 300 calories made up of carbohydrate (60%), protein (15%) and fat (25%). At every meal, the hydration needs must also be satisfied since dehydration and depletion of carbohydrates are limiting factors in long runs.

GOOD NUTRITION GUIDE

1. Eat high quality foods rich in nutrients to supply adequate calories. These should contain whole grains, cereals, fruits and vegetables, meat, fish or other protein sources and dairy products.

2. Complex carbohydrates (breads, pasta, rice, bagels) should form about 60 – 70 % of the total daily calories in a runner's diet.

3. 3 servings of vegetables and 2 servings of fruits daily should provide the needed vitamins, minerals, fibre and additional carbohydrates.

4. As for fats, aim for 10 - 20% of the total daily calories while simple sugars (from sweets, cakes, fruit drinks) should be less than 10%.

5. Eat regularly throughout the day and don't skip breakfast.

6. Eat the right kind of food before, during and after running.

7. For moderate intensity running of over 1 hr, take 15 g of carbohydrate 15 mins before, 20 g every 20 mins during the run and after the run, take 1.0-1.5 g/kg of carbohydrate and 0.1-0.2g/kg of protein to refuel.

NUTRITION FOR RACE DAY

1. For races longer than 10 km such as half-marathons and marathons, consume a high carbohydrate diet (pastas, bread, rice or potatoes) known as carbo loading, for a couple of days before the race to store enough glycogen for race day.

2. On race day, don't overload. Consume your usual breakfast, mostly complex carbohydrates (cereals, toasts, bagels and fruits for a total of about 150 grams) plus a little protein (from skim milk).

3. Avoid high-fat foods since they are hard to digest.

4. Don't try any new foods or drinks at this stage.

5. Allow 1-2 hours for the food to be fully digested to avoid possible stomach distress during the race.

6. Drink a cup of coffee or juice or water.

7. Consume 25 g of simple carbohydrate 15 minutes before the race starts to make sure your glycogen levels are topped up.

8. During the race, refuel every 20 minutes with a sports drink or if you prefer take a gel every hour with plenty of water.

9. Don't forget to refuel as soon as the race is over with 75g of carbohydrate and 10g of protein and a little bit of fat.

POST-RACE REFUELING

It is important to refuel the body as soon as the race is over, the priority being to replace the glycogen lost and to re-hydrate.

Use a high glucose drink (50 g) in the first 15 minutes after the race is over. It will be rapidly absorbed to refill the depleted glycogen stores and will also re-hydrate you at the same time. You could also have a sports drink (800 ml), fruit juice (500 ml), whole wheat cereal with milk (1 glass), fruit (3 pieces) or bread (2 slices) with jam. Include some protein to start the healing of damaged muscles.

Keep on eating every 30 minutes for another 2 hours (for a total of 100g) rather than taking one large meal as it increases glycogen absorption. ◆

FOOD 4 FAST FEET

71

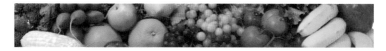

CHAPTER 11

MEAL IDEAS

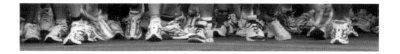

In this chapter, you will find ideas for breakfast, lunch, snacks and dinner for seven days of the week. The approximate carbohydrate, protein and fat contents of the food as well as the total calories are given alongside.

BREAKFASTS FOR 7 DAYS

Day 1 Breakfast

Cup of oatmeal cooked in ½ cup of milk sweetened with honey; two slices of whole wheat bread with two scoops of Becel margarine and jam; one cup of tea.

FOOD CALORIES	CARB/g	PRO/g	FAT/g	CAL/g
1 cup oatmeal	30	4	2	154
½ cup skim milk	5.0	3.4	0.1	34
1 tbsp honey	15	0	0	60
2 slices whole wheat bread	30	4..5	2.7	152
2 tsp. Becel margarine	0	0	3.5	31
1 tbsp jam	14	0.2	0	60
1 cup of tea	0	0.2	0	1
Total:	**94**	**12.3**	**8.3**	**492**

Day 2 Breakfast

One scrambled egg with one slice of tomato and grated cheddar (1 tbsp) and two slices of whole wheat toasts; one cup of coffee.

FOOD CALORIES	CARB/g	PRO/g	FAT/g	CAL/g
1 scrambled egg	0	10	23	250
1 tbsp grated cheddar	0.5	3	1.5	27
2 slices whole wheat toast	30	4.5	2.5	152
1 cup of black coffee	0	0.4	0	2
Total:	**30.5**	**17.9**	**27.2**	**431**

Day 3 Breakfast

Two pieces of toast with strawberry jam; ½ cup yogurt; cup of tea

FOOD CALORIES	CARB/g	PRO/g	FAT/g	CAL/g
2 slices of bread	30	4	2	154
1tbsp strawberry jam	14	0.2	0	60
1 cup low-fat fruit yoghurt	28	6	1	145
1 cup of tea	0	0.2	0	1
Total:	**72**	**10.4**	**3**	**359**

Day 4 Breakfast

One bagel with 2 tbsp peanut butter; 1 medium banana; 1 cup of coffee.

FOOD CALORIES	CARB/g	PRO/g	FAT/g	CAL/g
1 bagel (120 g)	55	11	2	282
2 tbsp peanut butter	6	8	16	200
1 medium banana	25	0	0	100
1 cup of coffee	0	0.4	0	2
Total:	**86**	**19.4**	**18**	**584**

Day 5 Breakfast

1 Cup of corn flakes, ½ cup milk and 1 tbsp honey; 2 pieces of toast with butter (1 tbsp) and jam (1 tbsp) ; 1 cup of coffee.

FOOD CALORIES	CARB/g	PRO/g	FAT/g	CAL/g
1 cup corn flakes	37	2	0	156
1 cup milk (1%)	12	9	2	102
1 tbsp honey	16	0	0	64
2 pieces of toast	32	7	2	174
2 tsp butter	0	0	10	90
1 tbsp jam	14	0	0	56
1 cup of coffee	0	0.4	0	2
Total:	**111**	**17.4**	**14**	**644**

Day 6 Breakfast

½ Cup granola with ½ cup yogurt and ½ cup of fruit salad; 2 pieces of toast with peanut butter (1 tbsp); 1 cup of green tea.

FOOD CALORIES	CARB/g	PRO/g	FAT/g	CAL/g
½ cup granola	36	5	6	218
1 cup yoghurt (0 fat)	25	8	0	132
½ cup fruit salad	15	0	0	60
2 pieces of toast	32	7	2	174
1 tbsp jam	15	0	0	60
1 cup green tea	0	0	0	0
Total:	**111**	**24**	**16**	**644**

Day 7 Breakfast

1 Cup of oatmeal with ½ cup of milk and two tbsp of raspberries;
1 poached egg with 2 pieces of toast; 1 glass orange juice

FOOD CALORIES		CARB/g	PRO/g	FAT/g	CAL/g
1 cup oatmeal		30	4	2	154
1 cup milk (1%)		12	9	2	102
½ cup raspberries		6	0	0	24
1 poached egg		0	6	5	69
2 pieces of toast		32	7	2	174
1 glass orange juice		30	0	0	120
	Total:	**110**	**25**	**11**	**643**

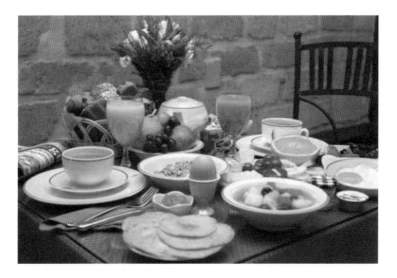

Healthy Breakfast for Two

LUNCHES FOR 7 DAYS

Day 1 Lunch

Roast turkey sandwich with multigrain bread, tomato, cucumber, lettuce and mayonnaise; 1 carrot muffin; 1 banana; 1 apple; 1 cup of coffee

FOOD CALORIES	CARB/g	PRO/g	FAT/g	CAL/g
roast turkey (50g)	0	14	2	74
2 slices multigrain bread	30	4	2	154
tomato, lettuce, cucumber	3	0	0	12
1 tbsp mayonnaise	0	0	5	45
1 carrot muffin	27	6	2	150
1 banana	25	0	0	100
1 apple	20	0	0	80
1 cup of coffee	0	0.4	0	2
Total:	**105**	**24.4**	**11**	**617**

Day 2 Lunch

1 Whole-wheat pita with canned salmon, red onions and tomato; 1 blueberry muffin; ½ avocado; 1 apple; 1 glass of milk

FOOD CALORIES	CARB/g	PRO/g	FAT/g	CAL/g
1 whole-wheat pita	29	6	1	149
canned salmon (50g)	0	10	4	76
red onions & tomato	2	0	0	8
1 blueberry muffin	32	6	1	161
½ avocado	0	0	15	135
1 apple	20	0	0	80
1 glass of milk(1%)	12	9	2	102
Total:	**95**	**31**	**23**	**711**

Day 3 Lunch

2 Pieces of toast with cheddar cheese and tomato; 2 chocolate chip cookies; half a cup of melon; 1 banana; 1 cup of green tea

FOOD CALORIES	CARB/g	PRO/g	FAT/g	CAL/g
2 pieces of toast	32	7	2	174
2 slices of cheddar	0	14	15	191
2 chocolate chip cookies	15	1	4	100
½ cup melon	8	0	0	32
1 banana	25	0	0	100
1 cup of green tea	0	0	0	0
Total:	80	22	21	597

Day 4 Lunch

Tuna salad with tomato, lettuce, beetroot with Italian dressing and 2 slices of whole-wheat bread; 1 low-fat fruit yogurt; 1 apple; 1 cup of chocolate milk

FOOD CALORIES	CARB/g	PRO/g	FAT/g	CAL/g
½ cup flaked tuna (50g)	0	12	1	57
tomato, lettuce, beetroot	3	0	0	12
1 tbsp dressing	0	0	5	45
2 slices of bread	30	6	2	162
1 fruit yogurt	25	8	0	132
1 apple	20	0	0	80
1 chocolate milk (8 oz)	26	8	8	208
Total:	104	34	15	696

Day 5 Lunch

1 Cup minestrone soup; 1 roast beef sandwich with Dijon mustard; fruit salad; 1 cup of coffee

FOOD CALORIES	CARB/g	PRO/g	FAT/g	CAL/g
1 cup minestrone soup	11	4	3	87
roast beef (100g)	0	25	4	136
2 slices whole wheat bread	30	6	2	162
Dijon mustard	0	0	0	0
fruit salad (1 cup)	30	0	0	120
1 cup coffee	0	0.4	0	2
Total:	**71**	**29.4**	**9**	**507**

Day 6 Lunch

2 Whole-wheat rolls with hummus; ¼ Honeydew melon; 1 fruit yogurt; 1 glass of chocolate milk

FOOD CALORIES	CARB/g	PRO/g	FAT/g	CAL/g
spicy hummus (4 tbsp)	6	2	6	86
2 whole-wheat rolls	30	6	2	162
¼ Honeydew melon	15	0	0	60
1 fruit yogurt (low-fat)	16	3	1.5	90
1 chocolate milk	26	8	8	208
Total:	**93**	**19**	**17.5**	**606**

Day 7 Lunch

1 Grilled chicken sandwich with lettuce, tomato, red onion and mayonnaise; 2 fig cookies; 1 banana; 1 glass of milk

FOOD CALORIES	CARB/g	PRO/g	FAT/g	CAL/g
grilled chicken (100g)	0	23	3.5	123
2 slices bread	30	6	2	162
3 tsp. butter (20g)	0	0	16	144
lettuce, tomato, red onion	2	0	0	8
mayonnaise (1 tbsp)	0	0	5	45
2 fig cookies	22	1	2	110
1 banana	25	0	0	100
1 glass milk (1%)	12	9	2	102
Total:	**80**	**39**	**30.5**	**794**

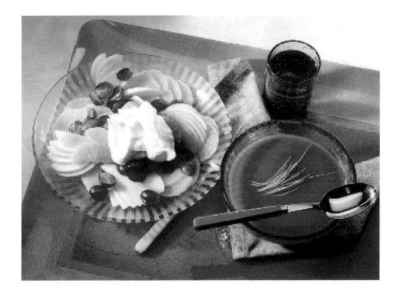

Healthy Lunch for One

DINNERS FOR 7 DAYS

Day 1 Dinner

1 cup minestrone soup; garlic bread (1 piece); red wine (1 glass); veggie pizza (1 slice); rhubarb tart (1 slice); cup green tea

FOOD CALORIES	CARB/g	PRO/g	FAT/g	CAL/g
Minestrone soup (1 cup)	11	4	3	87
Garlic bread (1 piece)	35	7	17	321
Vegetable pizza (1 slice)	27	9	5	189
Red wine (100 ml)	0	0	0	70
Rhubarb tart (1 slice)	25	1	6	158
Green tea (1 cup)	0	0	0	0
Total:	98	21	31	825

Day 2 Dinner

Lettuce salad with oil dressing (1 tbsp); grilled salmon; grilled mixed vegetables (1 cup); cooked couscous (1 cup); plum and oat crisp (1 slice); cup of coffee

FOOD CALORIES	CARB/g	PRO/g	FAT/g	CAL/g
Lettuce salad	2	0	0	8
Olive oil (1 tbsp)	0	0	9	81
Grilled salmon (100g)	0	23	10	182
Grilled mixed veg. (1 cup)	10	4	0	56
Cooked couscous (1 cup)	35	6	1	173
Plum & oat crisp (1 slice)	40	5	10	270
Cup of coffee	0	0.4	0	2
Total:	87	38.4	30	772

Day 3 Dinner

Caesar salad (1 cup); 100 g chicken in curry sauce (2 tbsp); Basmati rice (1/2 cup); 1 cup strawberries; ice milk (½ cup); cup of black tea

FOOD CALORIES	CARB/g	PRO/g	FAT/g	CAL/g
Caesar salad (1 cup)	10	5	13	177
Chicken (100g)	0	22	3	115
Curry sauce (2 tbsp)	6	1	6	82
Basmati rice (1/2 cup)	23	2.7	0	103
Strawberries (1 cup)	15	0	0	60
Ice milk (1 cup)	25	0	0	100
Cup black tea	0	0	0	0
Total:	**79**	**30.7**	**22**	**637**

Day 4 Dinner

Roast turkey (100g); boiled potatoes (50g); cooked Brussel sprouts (50g); boiled peas (50 g); lemon meringue pie (1 slice); glass of milk

FOOD CALORIES	CARB/g	PRO/g	FAT/g	CAL/g
Roast turkey (100g)	0	29	3	143
Boiled potatoes (50g)	19.7	1.4	0	84
Brussel sprouts (50g)	2	3	0	20
Boiled peas (50g)	4.3	5.4	0.4	42
Lemon meringue pie (1 slice)	76	4	12	428
Glass of skim milk (1 cup)	13	9	0	88
Total:	**115**	**52**	**15.4**	**805**

Day 5 Dinner

Lettuce, tomato salad; vinaigrette dressing (1 tbsp); 100g lemon sole fried in breadcrumbs; boiled cauliflower; potato baked in skin; slice of blueberry cobbler; cup of herbal tea

FOOD CALORIES	CARB/g	PRO/g	FAT/g	CAL/g
Lettuce and tomato salad	2	0	0	8
Vinaigrette dressing (1 tbsp)	0	0	9	81
Fried lemon sole (100g)	9	16	13	217
Boiled cauliflower (50g)	1	1.5	0	10
1 Potato baked in skin	20	2	0	88
Blueberry cobbler (1 slice)	46	4	7	263
Herbal tea (1 cup)	0	0	0	0
Total:	**77**	**23.5**	**29**	**667**

Day 6 Dinner

Tomato, cucumber salad with French dressing; 1cup whole wheat pasta; ½ cup tomato sauce; parmesan cheese (20g); strawberry shortcake (1 slice); glass of water.

FOOD CALORIES	CARB/g	PRO/g	FAT/g	CAL/g
Tomato, cucumber salad	3	0	0	12
French dressing (1 tbsp)	0	0	5	45
Whole wheat pasta (1 cup)	37	7	1	185
Tomato sauce (1/2 cup)	15	0	3	87
Parmesan cheese (40g)	0	14	12	164
Berry shortcake (1 slice)	49	5	10	306
Water (1 glass)	0	0	0	0
Total:	**104**	**26**	**31**	**799**

Day 7 Dinner

Lettuce, tomato, red peppers, red onion salad with oil and vinegar dressing (1 tbsp); grilled steak (100 g); roast potatoes (1/2 cup); boiled carrots (1/2 cup); cooked broccoli (1/2 cup); pear almond tart (1 slice); cup of tea.

FOOD CALORIES	CARB/g	PRO/g	FAT/g	CAL/g
Mixed lettuce salad	3	0	0	12
Oil & vinegar dressing (1 tbsp)	0	0	9	81
Grilled beef steak (100g)	0	27	12	216
Roast potatoes (1/2 cup)	30	3	6	186
Boiled carrots (1/2 cup)	5	2	0	28
Cooked broccoli (1/2 cup)	2	1	0	12
Pear almond tart (1 slice)	29	2	9	205
Cup of tea	0	0	0	0
Total:	**66**	**35**	**27**	**647**

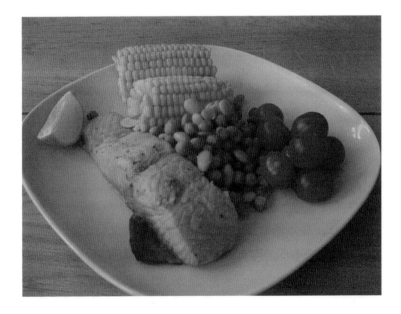

SNACKS

Snacks for eating 1 hour or less before exercising:

FOOD CALORIES	CARB/g	PRO/g	FAT/g	CAL/g
1 Apple	20	0	0	80
1 Orange	20	0	0	80
Grapes (1 cup)	25	1	0	104
Berries (1 cup)	15	0	0	60
Fruit salad (1 cup)	30	0	0	120
1 Banana	30	0	0	120
Vegetable soup (1 cup)	24	4	0	112
Carrots (100g)	5	1	0	24
Dates (50g)	27	1	0	112
Pure fruit juices (100g)	30	0	0	120
Raisins (100g)	65	1	0	264
1 Low-fat yoghurt	16	3	1.5	90
Gatorade (250 ml)	16	0	0	64
Toast (1 slice)+ jam (2 tsp)	29	3	0	128
Fig bars (2)	22	1	2	110
Sports gel (1 pack) + water	27	0	0	108
Powerade (170 ml)	41	0	0	164

Snacks for refueling after running (0 – 1 hour):

FOOD CALORIES	CARB/g	PRO/g	FAT/g	CAL/g
Skim milk (1 cup)	13	9	0	88
Chocolate milk 1% (1 cup)	26	9	2.5	163
Cheddar cheese (30g)	0	7	10	118
1 Plain bagel (125g)	60	12	2	306
Honey (1 tbsp)	17	0	0	68
Bread rolls (100g)	54	10	7	319
Almonds (25g)	1	4	14	146
Fruit cake (100g)	58	4	11	347
Porridge with bran (100g)	60	11	7	347
1 hard boiled egg	0	6	5	69
Bread (1 slice)+ peanut butter	18	7	8	172
Low-fat fruit yogurt (175g)	28	6	1	145
Chocolate chip cookie (17g)	17.5	1	4	110

MIXING AND MATCHING MENUS

As shown in *Chapter 4*, a *68 Kg/150 lb female* running for around 1.5 hours daily requires *2960 calories*. Her nutrient needs were calculated as follows:

From Table 4, carbohydrate required at 6g per kg of body weight:
$$68 \text{ kg} \times 6 = 408 \text{ g}$$

From Table 5, protein required at 1.6 g per kg of body weight:
$$68 \text{ kg} \times 1.6 = 109 \text{ g}$$

By adding the calories obtained from the carbohydrate and protein components of her diet and then subtracting it from the total calories required *(2960 calories)*, the calories from fat can be calculated. And since 1 gram of fat gives off 9 calories, the equivalent amount of fat is determined to be 99.1 grams.

So, the runner's daily intake should consist of the following:

	CARB/g	PRO/g	FAT/g	CAL/g
Target per day for Runner	408	109	99	2960

From the lists of breakfast, lunch and dinner menus as well as snacks, you can mix and match them in order to get the total daily calories appropriate for you. If you find that the total calories add up to more than what you need, simply omit one or more items from the various menus. *You could also split up items from the lunch menus and eat them as afternoon or evening snacks.* If, on the other hand, you need more calories, simply add more pre-run or post-run snacks. However, apart from total calories, *you should also ensure that you are getting adequate amounts of carbohydrate, protein and fat for someone running your mileage.*

ALLOCATION OF CALORIES DURING THE DAY

It is well known that to be fully energized all day long, one should eat frequently (also known as grazing), rather than eating all the calories in a couple of big meals.

The above 68 kg (150 lb) female runner can satisfy her nutritional requirements for one day, for example, by combining *Day 4 Breakfast, Day 6 Lunch,* and *Day 2 Dinner.* She also has to consume a sports drink during her morning run, snacks for recovery after the run as well as in the afternoon and evening. By spreading her calorie intake throughout the day, the runner will be well energized all day long.

FOOD CALORIES	CARB/g	PRO/g	FAT/g	CAL/g
1) Breakfast # 4 at 8am	86	19	18	584
2) Powerade during run 10am	41	0	0	164
3) Recovery snacks 11:30am				
Chocolate milk (360 ml)	39	12	12	312
Cheese (30 g)	0	7	10	118
4) Lunch # 6 at 1pm-2pm	93	19	18	606
5) Afternoon snacks at 5pm				
2 chocolate chip cookies	35	2	8	220
1 cup skim milk (250 ml)	12	9	0	84
6) Dinner # 2 at 7pm	87	38	30	772
8) Evening snack at 9pm				
Blueberry yogurt (100g)	15	4	3	103
Total:	**408**	**110**	**99**	**2963**

The food table below gives the number of calories, protein, fat and carbohydrate in *100 grams of some common food items.* Use it to add variations to your meals but always remember to check that you are meeting your nutrient and energy needs.

FOOD TABLE

FOOD/100 grams	ENERGY/cal	PRO/g	FAT/g	CARBS/g
All Bran	250	13	2.5	46
Almonds	560	17	54	4
Apples	35	0.2	0	9
Apricots	30	0.6	0	7
Artichokes boiled	15	1	0	3
Asparagus boiled	8.8	1.7	0	0.5
Aubergine raw	15	0.7	0	3
Avocados	220	4	20	2
Bacon gammon grilled	230	30	12	0
Bacon rashers streaky fried	500	23	45	0
Baked Beans - Heinz	74	5	0.3	12.7
Bananas	80	1	0.3	20
Bean sprouts canned	10	1.6	0	0.8
Beans broad boiled	50	4	0.6	7
Beans French boiled	7	0.8	0	1
Beef minced stewed	230	23	15	0
Beef rump steak fried	250	29	15	0
Beef rump steak grilled	220	27	12	0
Beef sirloin roast	280	24	21	0
Beef steak	220	30	11	0
Beef topside roast	200	27	12	0
Beer bitter	30	0	0	2
Beer stout	40	0	0	4
Beetroot boiled	45	1.8	0	10
Beetroot raw	30	1.3	0	6
Bilberries	60	0.5	0	14
Biscuits - morning coffee	444	6.9	14.5	75.4
Biscuits - Rich Tea	440	6.9	15.7	71.5
Biscuits water	440	11	12.5	76
Black Currants	30	1	0	7

FOOD/100 grams	ENERGY/cal	PRO/g	FAT/g	CARBS/g
Blackberries	30	1.5	0	6
Bran Flakes	329	9.3	2	71.5
Bran wheat	200	14	5.5	27
Brazil Nuts	600	12	60	4
Bread brown	220	9	2.2	45
Bread rolls white	300	10	7	54
Bread white	235	7.8	1.6	46.2
Bread white toasted	300	9.6	1.7	65
Broccoli tops boiled	20	3	0	1.6
Brussels sprouts boiled	20	3	0	1.7
Butter	750	0.5	82	0
Cabbage savoy boiled	10	1.3	0	1
Cabbage savoy raw	25	3	0	3
Cabbage spring boiled	8	1	0	1
Cabbage winter boiled	15	1.7	0	2.3
Cake fruit	330	4	11	58
Carrots boiled	20	0.6	0	4
Carrots raw	25	0.7	0	5
Cauliflower boiled	10	1.5	0	0.8
Cauliflower cheese	116	6	8	5
Celery raw	10	1	0	1.3
Cheese camembert	300	23	23	0
Cheese cheddar	400	26	34	0
Cheese cottage	66.5	14	0.5	1.5
Cheese cream	440	3	47	0
Cheese danish blue	360	23	29	0
Cheese edam	300	24	23	0
Cheese parmesan	400	35	30	0
Cherries	40	0.5	0	10
Chicken roast boned	150	25	5	0
Chicken roast meat	159	22	7.5	0
Chocolate milk	530	8	30	59
Chocolate plain	530	5	29	65
Christmas Pudding	300	5	12	48
Cocoa powder	300	19	22	12
Coconut desiccated	600	6	62	6
Cod fillet baked	100	21	1.2	0
Cod fillet fried	170	21	8	4
Cod fillet fried in batter	200	20	10	8

FOOD/100 grams	ENERGY/cal	PRO/g	FAT/g	CARBS/g
Cod fillet grilled	100	21	1.3	0
Cod fillet poached	90	21	1	0
Cod fillet steamed	80	19	1	0
Coke diet	0.48	0	0	0.12
Cornflakes	350	8	0.5	82
Crab canned	80	18	1	0
Cranberries	18	0.5	0	4
Cream single	200	2.4	21.2	3
Cream whipping	330	1.9	35	2.5
Crispbread rye	320	9.5	2	71
Crispbread wheat	390	45	7.5	37
Croissant	230	4.3	12.2	27.3
Cucumber	10	0.6	0	2
Currants dried	240	2	0	63
Dates dried	210	2	0	55
Drinking chocolate	370	6	6	77
Egg scrambled	250	10	23	0
Egg yolk	340	16.1	30.5	0
Eggwhite	35	9	0	0
Flour brown	330	13	2	69
Flour white	340	11	1.2	75
Flour white self raising	340	9	1.2	77.5
Flour wholemeal	320	13	2	66
Fruit gums	170	1	0	45
Fruit juice sweetened	40	0	0	10
Fruit juice unsweetened	30	0	0	8
Fruit pie	370	4	16	56
Fruit salad canned	101.2	0.3	0	25
Grapefruit peeled	20	0.5	0	5
Grapes black	50	0.5	0	13
Grapes white	60	0.6	0	15
Green Bean Mix	25.71	1.21	0.53	4.18
Halibut steamed	130	24	4	0
Ham cooked	269	24.7	18.9	0
Hamburgers fried	260	20	17	7
Honey	290	0	0	76
Ice cream dairy	170	4	7	25
Jams	260	0.5	0	60
Lamb leg roast	270	26	18	0

FOOD/100 grams	ENERGY/cal	PRO/g	FAT/g	CARBS/g
Leeks boiled	25	1.8	0	5
Lemon curd	280	0	5	63
Lemon juice	7.2	0.3	0	1.5
Lemon sole fried w/bcrumb	200	16	13	9
Lemon sole steamed	90	21	1	0
Lemonade bottled	24	0	0	6
Lemons	15	1	0	3
Lentils boiled	100	8	0.5	17
Lettuce	8	1	0	1
Luncheon meat	300	13	27	5
Macaroni boiled	120	4	0.6	25
Macaroni cheese - Tin	97	3.6	4.8	10.5
Mangoes	60	0.5	0	15
Macaroni cheese	170	7	10	15
Margarine	730	0	81	0
Margarine low fat spread	370	0	40	0
Marmalade	260	0	0	69
Mayonnaise	720	2	79	0
Melon	22	0.5	0	5
Milk	65	3.3	3.8	4.7
Milk skimmed	33	3.4	0.1	5
Mushrooms fried	210	2.2	22	0
Mushrooms raw	13.4	2	0.6	0
Oil vegetable	900	0	100	0
Omelet	200	11	16	0
Onions raw	25	1	0	5
Onions spring	35	1	0	8.5
Orange juice	40	0.6	0	9
Orange peeled	40	1	0	9
Pancakes	300	6	16	36
Pasta	365	13.2	2	77
Peaches canned	49	0.5	0	12.3
Peaches fresh	34	0.5	0	8
Peanuts fresh	570	24	50	9
Peanuts roasted and salted	570	24	50	9
Pears	30	0.2	0	8
Peas boiled	41	5.4	0.4	4.3
Peas canned	50	5	0.3	7
Peppers green raw	15	1	0.4	2

FOOD/100 grams	ENERGY/cal	PRO/g	FAT/g	CARBS/g
Pineapple fresh	50	0.5	0	12
Porridge Oats with Bran	332	10.6	6.7	60
Potato chips	250	4	11	37
Potato crisps	526	7.3	35.2	48.4
Potatoes baked with skin	85	2	0	20
Potatoes boiled	82	1.4	0.1	19.7
Prawns	100	23	2	0
Radish	15	1	0	3
Raisins	250	1	0	65
Raspberries	28	1	0	6
Rice Brown Boiled	182	3.4	1.4	40.7
Rice white boiled	119	2.6	0.1	28
Salad Cream	300	2	27	15
Salmon steamed	200	20	13	0
Sardines canned in oil	220	24	14	0
Sausages beef grilled	270	13	17	15
Sausages pork	320	13	25	12
Scones	370	7.5	15	56
Spaghetti boiled	120	4	0.3	26
Spring greens boiled	10	1.7	0	1
Strawberries fresh	25	0.5	0	6
Sugar	390	0	0	100
Sugar puffs cereal	350	6	0.8	84
Sultanas	250	2	0	65
Tangerines peeled	36	1	0	8
Toffees	430	2	17	71
Tomato juice	12	0	0	3
Tomato Ketchup	97	1	0	24.9
Tomatoes raw	15	1	0	3
Tuna canned in oil	100	25	0.1	0
Turkey roast	140	29	3	0
Walnuts	530	11	52	5
Wine red	70	0	0	0
Wine white dry	65	0	0	0.6
Yogurt flavoured - low fat	41.6	4.6	0.1	5.5
Yogurt natural	55	5.9	1.2	5.6

Adapted from a Food Table by A.E. Bender and D.A. Bender

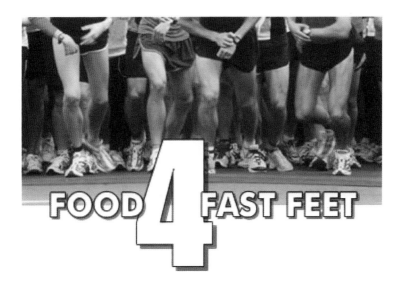

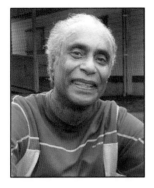

ABOUT THE AUTHOR

After spending 33 years as a Chemistry Lecturer at Montreal's Dawson College, John Abbott College and briefly, the Food Science Department of McGill University, Dr. Bala Naidoo retired in 2005 and settled down in Ladysmith, on Vancouver Island, British Columbia.

Dr. Bala Naidoo started running in the early seventies and has not stopped since! Both he and his wife Pauline are members of the Ladysmith Striders and they take part regularly in the Vancouver Island series of races.

Combining his passion for running with his long-standing interest in nutrition, has given rise to his new book, "Food 4 Fast Feet".

Dr. Bala Naidoo is the author of the following two books on nutrition:

Nature's Bounty: Why Certain Foods Are So Good For You (BookSurge, 2004)

Nature's Bounty: More About Foods For A Longer And Healthier Life (BookSurge, 2005)

Both books are available at www.amazon.com and other favourite retailers.

DR. BALA NAIDOO